Breakthrough   Miracles   Testimonies

Receiving Your Miracle Baby Now

MARGARET EMA

**The Working Document
[Breakthrough Series]**

"It is the truth you know that makes you free"

John 8:32

Dedication

I dedicate this Book to the Holy Spirit our only source of fruitfulness and to my friend and covenant partner Blessing Achonye my motivation for writing this book of testimonies.

You are a Fruitful Vine

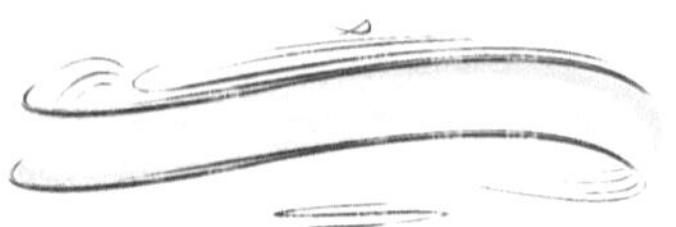

And the Lord Blessed them and said
"Be Fruitful and Multiply"
Genesis 1: 28

∞

Thus said the Lord
For I am the LORD, I change not; Malachi 3:6

∞

This is your Foundation and Assurance of Faith
Is anything too hard for the LORD?
At the time appointed I will return unto you,
according to the time of life, and Sarah [you] shall have a
son.
Gen 18: 14

∞

Behold, I am the LORD, the God of all flesh:
is there anything too hard for me?
Jeremiah 32: 27

∞

Jesus said unto him, if thou canst believe,
all things are possible to him that believes.
Mark 9: 23

∞

Jesus said unto her, Said I not unto you,
that, if you would believe,
you should see the glory of God?
John 11: 40

∞

Jesus said, the things which are impossible with men are
possible with God.
Luke 18:27

∞

*Now you must take these Scriptures and meditate on them –
and see God Almighty talking personally to you through
them.*

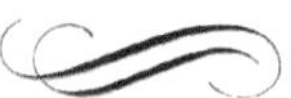

*"If the unbeliever - that is one not in Christ can walk in the bless-
ing and are fruitful and multiplying with children, how much
more the one that belongs to Christ and is a carrier of a more*

perfect blessing that is bought with the precious Blood of the Lamb of God. Think about this".

"God did not suggest that we "be fruitful and multiply and replenish the earth, it is a command. We are instructed by God to be productive; we are under command to reproduce after our own Kind".

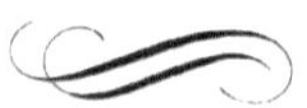

Contents

INTRODUCTION

From my heart to you,

Your Vision: what do you see?

Because what you see you cannot doubt and what you believe, you are supernaturally enabled to become. John 1: 12

Now below is the future that God has for you. I want you to spend time on this prophecy and allow this vision to give you a mental picture of your future.

See yourself as God sees you now. Let this become your reality, meditate on this truth until it becomes flesh and you become one with it.

Your wife shall be as a fruitful vine by the sides of your house: your children like olive plants round about your table.

Psalms 128:3

Lo, children are an heritage of the LORD: and the fruit of the womb is his reward.

4 As arrows are in the hand of a mighty man; so are children of the youth.

5 Happy is the man that hath his quiver full of them:
they shall not be ashamed, but they shall speak with
the enemies in the gate.

Psalm 127: 3 – 5

When you can see this vision, it will do something very powerful in you. I just want to warn you
so you will not become confused and allow the enemy to steal your victory:

- This book will <u>birth faith in your heart</u> – and
  you need faith to take delivery of the promise
  from God.

Margaret Ema

"Contrary to some opinion that some kind of affliction comes from God to teach us lessons; how can God partner with the devil to afflict his one of children and then partner with His Son Jesus to heal and deliver another. Then His Kingdom will certainly be divided against itself."

1

Can you see the Promise?

God made a promise to Abraham to give Him a child even though He was advanced in age.

After a while in Genesis chapter 15, Abraham sort of reminds God that he was still waiting for the fulfilment of this promise.

The response of the Lord is very interesting. God caused Abraham to see the picture of that promised future. It is at this point that Abraham settled in His heart that God was able and committed to do for him what He had promised.

He could see the future that God made him to see.

And He took him outside and said, "Now look toward the heavens, and count the stars, if you are able to count them." And He said to him, "So shall your descendants be."

6 Then he believed in the Lord; and He reckoned it to him as righteousness.

Genesis 15: 5 – 6

After seeing this picture of the future that God had planned for him because of the promised seed, Abraham believed God and it became his seal of faith.

A guarantee that surely, that child will become a reality because of the great future that God had attached to it. Has God said anything to you concerning your desire to have children?

Maybe not personally, but have you seen any of the promises that He has made that guarantees your fruitfulness which results in having Children?

If not, then the very purpose of this book is to show you the future that God has planned for you. Now, on the other hand, if you have received the word of the Lord, if you are standing on the promise of fruitfulness as the one we have as our foundation in this introduction, Psalm 127: 3 and Psalm 127: 3 – 5.

Then look at this again and see yourself exactly as God has said in that Scripture. Become fully persuaded in your heart that if you will believe, then God is committed to bring His Word to pass for you.

You may wonder if you must wait for such a long time like Abraham did, no you do not have to.

Jesus said that "it is unto you according to your faith" meaning that as you choose to believe God [you see to believe God and His Word is a choice, because faith is not passive, it is a conscious act based on the integrity of God's Word]

You activate the power of God to do what you want as you believe. Remember three fundamental truths about faith on this side of Salvation. Keep this in mind that:

1. Faith is now! Hebrews 11: 1

2. Now is the acceptable time for God to hear you

3. And **now** is the time of God's favour. 2 Corinthians 6: 2 NIV

You determine what you want and how and when you want it by choosing to believe God and His Word. We have a few Scriptural testimonies to prove this.

Faith is now; when you believe God completely regardless of contrary circumstance, His power is released to work on your behalf to hand you the promise.

We will see why Abraham experienced delay as we progress in this book.

Now meditate on the scriptures that shows you the plan of God for your fruitfulness and it will begin to show you your future. And as you see yourself in that future, it will become difficult to doubt God and your desire will certainly come.

The Word of God will show you the picture of your future and faith will bring it into your today.

A dear servant of God often says that "what you see, you cannot doubt" how true. I urge you to please open your heart and believe God now. May God bless you and help your faith as you read, in the wonderful name of our Lord Jesus Christ. Your friend in Christ

"The Father sent His Son to come and connect us back to His plan which is the blessing – that through Jesus Christ "<u>all the families of the earth be blessed</u>" in deed"

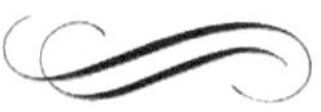

2

God's Plan is still the Blessing

God's plan is always the blessing

*I*n every dispensation, every generation, and every new beginning, God speaks the blessing over someone and that blessing is pronounced over all of humanity.

Let's see a few examples that show us this truth; First God reveals to us His plan for mankind – which is the Blessing.

Adam and Eve

And God blessed them, and God said unto them, be fruitful, and multiply, and replenish the earth, and subdue it: and have dominion over the fish of the sea, and over the fowl of the air, and over every living thing that moves upon the earth.
Genesis 1: 28

It is important to note at this point that God did not pronounce the blessing until He had created Eve and brought the man and woman into the union of marriage.

Adam was created a while before Eve.

We have no idea how long Adam spent in the garden alone before God made the statement that "it is not good for man to be alone"

But it is only after the union of marriage was instituted that "the Blessing" was pronounced and God gave the instruction or command to them and said;

"Be fruitful and multiply and replenish the earth"

You see this is the plan of God for every union of marriage and this plan has not changed!

Provision for food as part of the blessing

And God said, Behold, I have given you every herb bearing seed, which is upon the face of all the earth, and every tree, in the which is the fruit of a tree yielding seed; to you it shall be for meat.

30 And to every beast of the earth, and to every fowl of the air, and to everything that creeps upon the earth, wherein there is life, I have given every green herb for meat: and it was so.

31 And God saw everything that he had made, and, behold, it was very good. And the evening and the morning were the sixth day.

Genesis 1:29 - 31

Noah

And God spoke unto Noah, saying, 16 Go forth of the ark, thou, and thy wife, and thy sons, and thy sons' wives with thee. 17 Bring forth with thee every living thing that is with thee, of all flesh, both of fowl, and of cattle, and of every creeping thing that creeps upon the earth; <u>that they may breed abundantly in the earth,</u> <u>and be fruitful, and multiply upon the earth.</u>

Genesis 8: 15 - 17

Abraham

Now the LORD had said unto Abram, get thee out of thy country, and from thy kindred, and from thy father's house, unto a land that I will show thee: 2 And I will make of thee a great nation, and I will bless thee, and make thy name great; and thou shalt be a blessing: 3 And I will bless them that bless thee, and curse him that curses thee: <u>and in thee shall all families of the earth be blessed</u>.

Genesis 12: 1 – 3

God's sworn Blessing on Abraham

And said, by myself have I sworn, said the LORD, for because thou hast done this thing, and hast not withheld thy son, your only son:

17 That in blessing I will bless thee, and in multiplying I will multiply thy seed as the stars of the heaven, and as the sand which is upon the sea shore; and thy seed shall possess the gate of his enemies;

18 <u>And in thy seed, shall all the nations of the earth be blessed</u>; because thou hast obeyed my voice.

Genesis 22: 16 - 18

Isaac

And the LORD appeared unto him, and said, Go not down into Egypt; dwell in the land which I shall tell thee of: 3 Sojourn in this land, and I will be with thee, and will bless thee; for unto thee, and unto thy seed, I will give all these countries, and I will perform the oath which I swore unto Abraham thy father; 4 And I will make thy seed to multiply as the stars of heaven, and will give unto thy seed all these countries; <u>and in thy seed shall all the nations of the earth be blessed</u>; 5 Because that Abraham obeyed my voice, and kept my charge, my commandments, my statutes, and my laws.

Genesis 26: 2 - 5

Jacob

I am the LORD God of Abraham thy father, and the God of Isaac: the land whereon thou lie, to thee will I give it, and to thy seed; 14 And thy seed shall be as the dust of the earth, and thou shalt spread abroad to the west, and to the east, and to the north, and to the south: <u>and in thee and in thy seed, shall all the families of the earth be blessed</u>.

Genesis 28: 13 – 14

What does it mean to be blessed, and what does blessing mean?

To Bless

1. To pronounce a wish of happiness to one; to express a wish or desire of happiness.

2. To make happy; to make successful; to prosper in temporal concerns; as, we are blest with peace and plenty.

To be Blessed

Participle present tense: Made happy or prosperous; extolled; pronounced happy.

Adjective: Happy; prosperous in worldly affairs; enjoying spiritual happiness and the favour of God; enjoying heavenly felicity.

Blessing

Participle present tense: Making happy; wishing happiness to; praising or extolling; consecrating by prayer.

Noun: Benediction; a wish of happiness pronounced; a prayer imploring happiness upon another.

1. A solemn prophetic benediction, in which happiness is desired, invoked or foretold.

2. Any means of happiness; a gift, benefit or advantage; that which promotes temporal prosperity and welfare, or secures immortal felicity. The divine favour is the greatest blessing

3. Among the Jews, a present; a gift; either because it was attended with kind wishes for the welfare of the giver, or because it was the means of increasing happiness.

The mind of God is revealed to us

The mind of God for man is revealed to us from Scripture. God wanted man blessed.

That means; to be happy, prosperous, productive, fruitful, successful secure, etc. and through the ages in- spite of all the disruption because of the fall of man and the introduction of sin.

God through the ages kept pronouncing the blessing on mankind as we have seen.

At every opportunity, God speaks a blessing that will cover all of humanity. God has not changed His mind about what He wants for man.

In-spite of sin, man is still productive, successful, fruitful and still replenishing the earth.

Now we are going to reveal the mind of God to bless all of mankind and how that has been sealed eternally in His Son Jesus Christ for as many as will believe.

We have seen conclusively that God's plan for you and for me is that we are blessed resulting in a fruitful and productive life.

The blessing makes one fruitful, productive and prosperous; and to be blessed means;

- Peace
- Happy
- Prosperous
- Productive

- Fruitful
- Successful
- Secure, life and so much more.

Each aspect of the blessing broken down here covers every area of our life.

We will look at the main ingredient of the blessing which is peace at a later Chapter. Peace is a sum of all the blessing.

Now we must understand that this does not only translate to being fruitful in having children, this means to be "blessed" in every way.

It means a "Shalom" life: which is to live a peaceful, content and fulfilled life. A life that is complete, a rich full life, and living life in abundance.

This is not in the future, this is for us now. Jesus has paid the price for us to live in the blessing now in this life time.

God's eternal plan for all of mankind is the blessing

Our Lord Jesus Christ
Now God consistently pronounced the blessing all through the ages until He delivered to us the

main source of the blessing which is through His Son Jesus Christ.

This is where God puts an eternal seal to His plan for mankind to be blessed. This is a plan for us to live a prosperous and full life; which is to have and live life in abundance.

God pronounced the blessing on Abraham, Isaac and Jacob in their generations. One thing consistent within the blessing is that, He always said "and in you and in your seed, shall all the families of the earth be blessed"

Jesus Christ is that promised seed that was to come and restore and establish the blessing as God's original intent for all of mankind.

Jesus is that promised seed that would come from the loins of Abraham through his Son Isaac and Jacob and their generations. The Scripture confirming this says;

Ye are the children of the prophets, and of the covenant which God made with our fathers, saying unto Abraham, and in thy seed, shall all the kindred of the earth be blessed. 26 Unto you first God, having raised up his Son Jesus, sent him to bless you, in turning away every one of you from his iniquities.

Acts 3: 25 – 26

Now to Abraham and his seed were the promises made. He said not, and to seeds, as of many; but as of one, and to thy seed, which is Christ.

Galatians 3:16

We belong in the generation of our Lord Jesus Christ and He is that promised seed that God spoke of to the Fathers Abraham, Isaac and Jacob.

Jesus is that seed that carries the blessing through whom all the nations of the earth are blessed.

He came to restore all things back to God and establish the plan of God and He accomplished that at a cost.

He paid a High price to restore the blessing to all mankind by a covenant relationship which is sealed with His own blood.

The Scripture said this of Him:

Yet it was the will of the Lord to bruise Him; He has put Him to grief and made Him sick. When You and He make His life an offering for sin [and He has risen from the dead, in time to come], He shall see His [spiritual] offspring, He shall prolong His days, <u>and the will and pleasure of the Lord shall prosper in His hand.</u>

Isaiah 53: 19

The Father sent His Son to come and connect us back to His plan which is the blessing.

That through Jesus Christ "<u>all the families of the earth be blessed</u>" in deed.

The Riches of Redemption

Now let me show you all the riches of redemption that is available to us now through Christ Jesus, we must believe and receive it, because this is what came with your Salvation package if you are saved.

Saying with a loud voice, worthy is the Lamb that was slain to receive **power**, and **riches**, and **wisdom**, and **strength**, and **honour**, and **glory**, and **blessing.**
Revelation 5:12

Now the power of "the Blessing" which is our focus in this book only makes up a portion of the total package that Salvation has brought us.

So even the unsaved sinner is still living and walking in the benefits of "the Blessing" that God pronounced upon man in the Garden of Eden.

To Noah after the flood, with sin still in the life of man, God spoke the blessing again and instructed man to be fruitful and multiply and replenish the earth.

If the unbeliever, the one who is not in Christ can walk in the blessing and multiply and are fruitful with children, how much more the one that belongs to Christ and is a carrier of a perfect blessing that is bought with the precious Blood of the Lamb of God. Think about this.

With Jesus came, the full weight of God's plan for us which now includes the Blessing, an empowerment, a supernatural ability to accomplish mighty things which includes fruitfulness and the ability to have children and dominion and authority on earth.

If an unbeliever can have children because of that instruction from the mouth of God in the garden of Eden to Adam and Eve "be fruitful and multiply" without even knowing the truth about it, if a person willingly living and practicing sin can be fruitful and multiply, how much more you who is blood bought, washed, and has been justified, sanctified, and made right with God how much more you.

Receive this truth today, let it persuade your heart about your rights in God to have children, and surely as God lives, no matter what the case is

the blessing will supply the ability for you to conceive and bring forth as many children as you desire. In the wonderful name of our Lord Jesus Christ! Amen

This chapter has laid a foundation for our faith as believers to the right to have children according to the will and plan of God; Faith will come to you now, for;

"by faith Sarah received strength to conceive seed, for she judged God faithful who has promised"

So, by Faith you will receive the supernatural ability to conceive seed and bring forth now. To the Glory of God forever!

What the rest of this book will do is persuade your heart to believe that you too can become a joyful mother and Father of children as God has purposed for you.

These chapters will build your faith in God and prepare you to take delivery of what is rightfully yours in God through His Son Jesus Christ.

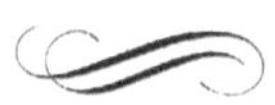

3

And the Lord Blessed them

G od created man in his own image, in the image of God created he him; male and female created he them. 28 And God blessed them, and God said unto them, be fruitful, and multiply, and replenish the earth, and subdue it: and have dominion over the fish of the sea, and over the fowl of the air, and over every living thing that move upon the earth.

Genesis 1: 27 – 28

R ight there is the plan of God for us, and we have said that this plan has not changed. We have seen that it is even made more secure by Redemption through Christ Jesus and it will always remain the plan of God for mankind.

God did not change His mind about anything that He declared and created in the Garden of Eden just because man fell and gave up His authority and dominion to the devil.

The temptation of Adam did not take God by surprise either.

The Scripture says that the Lamb of God was slain "from the foundation of the Word" Revelation 13: 8, therefore even before the fall of man, the plan of redemption was already in place.

This means that all through the process of creation, God knew that the devil would attempt and temporarily succeed to disrupt the plan of God for mankind whom God created in His own image and likeness to have dominion over all that God created.

Notice that even though the ground was cursed for Adam's sake and man was sent out of the Garden of the Lord, in Genesis Chapter 8 - after the flood of Noah, God spoke the same blessing again upon man and lifted the curse on the ground so that man will no longer have to toil to eat and be sustained.

God said, "I will not again curse the ground any more for man's sake" Genesis 8: 21

God spoke the Blessing again

And God spoke unto Noah, saying, 16 Go forth of the ark, thou, and thy wife, and thy sons, and thy sons' wives with thee. 17 Bring forth with thee every living thing that is with thee, of all flesh, both of fowl, and of cattle, and of every creeping thing that creeps upon the earth; that they may breed abundantly in the earth, and be fruitful, and multiply upon the earth.

Genesis 8: 15 – 17

The Blessing remains the heart and mind of God for all and He has not changed. He knew what He wanted from the beginning and nothing can change that.

It is important that we know this because it will help our faith.

Faith is the only way to receive from God. Faith is our Redemptive access to our rich heritage in Christ.

"Did you know that the temptation and fall of Adam

did not take God by surprise?"

Think about that!

4

Be Fruitful – It is a Command

Notice that God did not suggest that we "be fruitful and multiply and replenish the earth" it is a command. We are instructed by God to be productive; we are under command to reproduce after our own Kind.

God will not tell us to do what is impossible for us to do, that would be unjust. And the Scripture says that "His commandments are not gracious" that means; God's commands are not "burdensome" and impossible to accomplish. 1 John 5: 3

God commanded man to "be fruitful and multiply" when man was created and there was no sin in him and then again, we see God pronounce the same blessing again in Genesis chapter 8.

He commands man to "be fruitful and multiply" even after sin came and reigned which resulted in the flood of Noah, after the flood man was still in a state of sin because Jesus was not yet manifest. So even with sin, God still blessed man and told man to "be fruitful and multiply"

If you look at this two occasions, you will understand that in-spite of what the state of man is, God's command is still in force and it stands till today.

God is still saying to you right now in spite of what the Doctors have said, and in spite of how you feel, He is saying to you now "be fruitful and multiply and replenish the earth"

When God speaks everything else must obey. Your body must obey, your mind must obey. As hear the voice of God's Word today as He commands you to "be fruitful and multiply" Keep this instruction and command of Scripture in front of you with the full intention to obey and do what you are told.

Which is that you "be fruitful and multiply and replenish the earth"

Keep saying this to yourself and to your body until you are fully persuaded and yield yourself completely to God.

When God Speaks, His Word contains everything that is required to bring that Word to pass so all you need to do is to believe and act your faith by saying what you believe until you can see it then it will become yours, and it will be delivered to you.

God changed Abraham's name from Abram to Abraham declaring repeatedly as His name was continually called, from exalted "Father" to "The Father of many nations"

His testimony was being declared even before His Isaac came. keep announcing to yourself and your body that you are "fruitful and you multiply" in obedience to the instruction of the Lord!

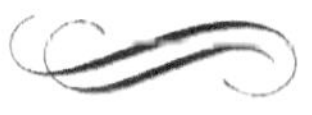

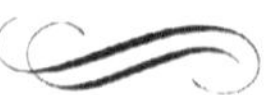

When God speaks everything else must obey, your body must obey, your mind must obey, so hear the voice of God's Word today as He commands you to "be fruitful and multiply"

" Keep this instruction and command of Scripture in front of you with the full intention to obey and do what you are told"

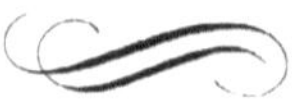

5

The Curse of Sin

Corruption came the day that man submitted his authority to the devil, from then on sin was introduced into man.

Sickness and disease came, compromise came, and wickedness and every evil work became part of the human existence.

Even though the kingdom of darkness right now is working against God and His purpose for man in this present world system, the plan of God is still in place whether we believe it or not.

The Word of God is a sworn oath, it is unchanging and incorruptible.

The LORD of hosts hath sworn, saying, surely as I have thought, so shall it come to pass; and as I have purposed, so shall it stand:

27 For the LORD of hosts has purposed, and who shall disannul it? And his hand is stretched out, and who shall turn it back?

Isaiah 14: 24 and 27

The Word of God is the only thing that the enemy cannot corrupt and the Scripture says that "we are born again of an incorruptible seed, the Word of God which lives and abides forever" 1 Peter 1: 23

If you are a believer, then you are born or the Word of God and will certainly live and be sustained by the Word of God only.

You must come to understand this, everything that God has for you is in His Word and can only come to you by faith as you believe. Your Children and your money are all in the Word of God, so do you believe it?

The Lord upholds all things by the Word of His power, The Word will not return to God void without accomplishing what God sent it to do.

Our Lord Jesus Christ said that Heaven and earth will pass away, but the Word abides forever. Matthew 24: 35, Mark 13: 31, Luke 21: 33

What this all points to, is the truth that even in the fallen state of man, the Word of God still stands firm. After all Adam and Eve were still fruitful and multiplied to replenish the earth even with a sin nature.

We are not upholding the state of sin here but rather we are enforcing the infallible nature and the power of God's Word. If you can believe the Word of God, then that Word will without fail produce in your life.

We went astray

Now we will look at some of the reason why mankind has experienced barrenness or delay in being fruitful and multiplying.

The Psalmist said, "before I was afflicted, I went astray" Psalm 119: 67.

Sometimes a person's life style can alter the natural reproductive system and bring about a lack of fruitfulness.

In this situation, as a believer there is healing and deliverance and there is recovery and restoration if we will accept the work of Salvation and repent of any kind of sin and turn to God, then such a person will certainly find mercy, because there is always mercy in God. It is all in the Word of God.

> He sent his word, and healed them, and delivered them from their destructions.

Psalms 107:20

An enemy has done this

Jesus explaining the parable of the tares said, "an enemy has done this" and the Scripture says in Acts 10:38 "how God anointed Jesus Christ of Nazareth with the Holy Ghost and with power who went about doing good, healing all that were oppressed of the devil, for God was with Him"

This Scripture is showing us the source of every kind of affliction and oppression. Contrary to some opinion that some affliction comes from God to teach us lessons; how can God partner with the devil to afflict one and then partner with His Son Jesus to heal and deliver another. Then His Kingdom will certainly be divided against itself.

Every kind of affliction has its root and source in sin and satanic oppression. Jesus declared to us His mission and that of the devil all in one verse of

Scripture and this reveals the mind of God towards us and points to the very source of evil and affliction of any kind.

> The thief cometh not, but for to steal, and to kill, and to destroy: I am come that they might have life, and that they might have it more abundantly.
>
> John 10:10

Sin which results in sickness and disease, affliction and unfruitfulness are all a by-product of the devil's mission to "kill, steal and to destroy" But we have the answer to that straight away from the same portion of Scripture and it is clearly put down for us, which is that "Jesus came to give us life, that we may have life more abundantly"

Make this Scripture the one Word from God that answers all your questions in life and you will see things turn and align with the plan and purpose of God for you, this is all because it is the very heart and mind of God for us in Christ Jesus.

Jesus came to

- **To give us life, so that we have it in abundance. John 10: 10**

-   To do good, to heal and deliver from every satanic oppression.
    Acts 10: 38

-   To destroy the Works of the devil.
    1 John 3:8

-   To connect us to the blessing
    Galatians 3: 14 Revelation 5: 12

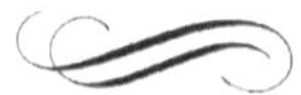

6

The Covenant Blessing

You are a seed of Abraham

At every stage that God finds a faithful man, He swears a blessing on Him and through that man the blessing is pronounce on mankind again, showing us that God's ultimate desire is that man be blessed, and be fruitful and multiply.

This time God introduced Himself to a man who was a heathen, an idol worshiper who did not know God, Abram, and gave him instructions to depart from His nation and kindred to a place God would show him.

Abraham obeyed and then God proclaims the blessing on him and said that through him and through His seed [Jesus Christ] the nations will be blessed.

> Now the LORD had said unto Abram, get thee out of thy country, and from thy kindred, and from thy father's house, unto a land that I will show thee: 2 And I will make of thee a great nation, and I will bless thee, and make thy name great; and thou shalt be a blessing: 3 And I will bless them that bless thee, and curse him that curse thee: and in thee shall all families of the earth be blessed.
>
> Genesis 12: 1 – 3

We continue to see the mind of God revealed to us, and in the midst of every declaration of "the blessing" is Jesus Christ who is the promised seed to Abraham through whom the nations of the earth will be blessed.

Now in Genesis 22 God brings the declaration of the blessing into a covenant relationship with Abraham still connecting "the blessing" now on the platform of the Covenant to all of mankind, we saw all of this in chapter one, but for emphasis He said:

And the angel of the LORD called unto Abraham out of heaven the second time, 16 And said, by myself have I sworn, said the LORD, for because thou hast done this thing, and hast not withheld thy son, your only son:

<u>That in blessing I will bless thee, and in multiplying I will multiply thy seed as the stars of the heaven, and as the sand which is upon the sea shore; and thy seed shall possess the gate of his enemies; 18 And in thy seed, shall all the nations of the earth be blessed;</u> because thou hast obeyed my voice.

Genesis 22: 16 - 18

The seed that carried the blessing referred to here was not Isaac but Jesus Christ.

This is confirmed to us In Galatians 3:16 -

"Now to Abraham and his seed were the promises made. He said not, and to seeds, as of many; but as of one, and to thy seed, which is Christ"

Now this is our connection to the blessing through our Lord Jesus Christ. Let us look further into this connection.

That the blessing of Abraham might come on the Gentiles through Jesus Christ; that we might receive the promise of the Spirit through faith.

And if ye be Christ's, then are ye Abraham's seed, and heirs according to the promise.

Galatians 3: 13 and 29

Through Christ Jesus we have become full beneficiaries of "the blessing" on this side of Salvation. This is the fulfilment of the plan of God to bless man which results in fruitfulness and multiplication. The Blessing and the command to "be fruitful and multiply" and replenish the earth is fulfilled in our lives as our heritage in Christ Jesus.

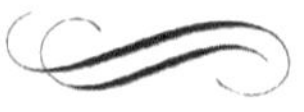

7

The Blessing and the Promised Seed

Our example

We are told to look to Abraham and to Sarah as our examples of faith in God and the example of God's commitment to His covenant relationship to Abraham. We will come to understand how to put our trust in God and how we can receive from God without having to wait as long as Abraham and Sarah had to wait before Isaac came.

Hearken to me, ye that follow after righteousness, ye that seek the LORD: look unto the rock whence ye are hewn, and to the hole of the pit whence ye are digged.

Look unto Abraham your father, and unto Sarah that bare you: for I called him alone, and blessed him, and increased him.

For the LORD shall comfort Zion: he will comfort all her waste places; and he will make her wilderness like Eden, and her desert like the garden of the LORD; joy and gladness shall be found therein, thanksgiving, and the voice of melody.

Isaiah 51: 1 - 3

God called Abraham and blessed him and made a promise to make him a blessing and through him and in his seed the nations of the earth will be blessed.

At this point, Abram and Sarai his wife had no children; Sarai was already called barren before now because they were already advanced in age.

Abram was seventy-five years and Sarai was in her sixties but God made a promise to bless them with a child.

The Promise

And the LORD appeared unto Abram, and said, unto thy seed will I give this land: and there built he an altar unto the LORD, who appeared unto him. Genesis 12: 7

And Abram said, Lord GOD, what wilt thou give me, seeing I go childless, and the steward of my house is this Eliezer of Damascus?

3 And Abram said, Behold, to me thou hast given no seed: and, lo, one born in my house is mine heir.

4 And, behold, the word of the LORD came unto him, saying, this shall not be your heir; but he that shall come forth out of your own bowels shall be your heir.

5 And he brought him forth abroad, and said, look now toward heaven, and tell the stars, if thou be able to number them: and he said unto him, so shall thy seed be. 6 And he believed in the LORD; and he counted it to him for righteousness.

Genesis 15: 2 – 6

Two things I want us to pay close attention to at this point is where the faith of Abram and Sarai his wife was at the time that God made the promise to give them an heir.

This will help us to understand how to position rightly to see prophecy fulfilled.

Abraham believed God

He was fully persuaded: Notice that at every given time that God made a promise to Abraham even the very first time when he did not know God and God just appeared to him and gave him instruction in Genesis twelve to leave his family and kinsfolk to an unknown destination,

Abram simply trusted and believed God and immediately took his family and left not knowing where he was headed for.

That is outstanding; to simply trust a God you do not know and have a relationship with.

To abandon all and put your future in the hand of an unknown God is commendable and yet most of us have come to know God for years and years and it will take so much for us to believe God let alone take a step of faith on the grounds of His Word only.

We may not hear God's audible voice, but His Word is "a more sure Word of prophecy" more sure and trusted than an audible voice of God. 2 Peter 1: 19

We are instructed to pay close attention to it as our light in that dark place in life until the breaking forth of dawn when the Word becomes fulfilled for us, the Word of God will give you light so that you can stand until you receive what you have believed God for.

Abraham was fully persuaded

The Scripture says that Abraham was fully persuaded that the God that made the promise had what it took to bring it to pass. He trusted God without any kind doubt.

This is how the Scripture puts it:

The Promise: (As it is written, I have made thee a father of many nations,) before him whom he believed, even God, who quickens the dead, and calls those things which be not as though they were.

Abraham believed God: Who against hope believed in hope, that he might become the father of many nations, according to that which was spoken, So shall thy seed be. 19 And being not weak in faith,

The prevailing circumstance not withstanding: He considered not his own body now dead, when he was about an hundred years old, neither yet the deadness of Sara's womb:

He did not doubt but gave God the Glory: He staggered not at the promise of God through unbelief; but was strong in faith, giving glory to God;

He was persuaded: And being fully persuaded that, what he had promised, he was able also to perform. 22 And therefore it was imputed to him for righteousness.

Romans 4: 17 - 22

Abraham had a conviction that God could be trusted; he had confidence in the integrity of the God who had made the promise.

Notice that God did not particularly go out of His way to convince Abraham to believe. All that God did was to make the promise and Abraham simply believed God and it was counted to him for righteousness.

Our ability to believe God, our faith in God and in His Word immediately puts us in right standing with God and positions us to receive from Him – to see His Word fulfilled for us.

Sarah had to Judged God faithful

Now on the other hand we will see the other side of things, you may be wondering that you do not have twenty five years to wait like Abraham did.

But you do not have to.

Something kept the promise from manifesting as quickly as Abraham believed God for it.

Sarah did not believe God as instantly as Abraham did, we see this as she persuades her husband to take her maid to wife to give him a son.

You can't really blame her, it had ceased to be with her after the manner of women and so physically she knew how impossible the promise was.

They were both advanced in age, but Abraham could still make children if he wanted as we saw with Sarah's maid Hagar.

Sarah was already bearing the reproach of barrenness even before they left their homeland Haran.

So that reality was very tangible to her which stood in the way of her ability to simply believe God.

You see, God did not just promise to give Abraham a son, but Sarah was an integral part of that promise.

The child had to come from Sarah who had long passed child bearing age.

Now think about that.

How Sarah came to believe – "she judged God faithful"

God needed Sarah's faith as well as Abraham, He needed her to believe and come into agreement with her husband for the promise to become manifest for them.

Our God only operates by faith and Sarah's faith was required to birth Isaac. Now Hebrews 11: 11 tell us how things changed and made it possible for the promised seed to be born. Let's see:

> Through faith also Sara herself received strength to conceive seed, and was delivered of a child when she

was past age, because she judged him faithful who had promised.

Hebrews 11:11

It took many years and the birth of Ismael and the appearance to an Angel of God to bring Sarah to the place where she eventually understood and came to terms with the truth that God meant exactly what He had said about giving Abraham a son through her.

Even when the Angel came, Sarah laughed at God mockingly, that is why God was angry with her and rebuked her. It was at this point that she settled down to "Judge God" another translation says that she "considered" God faithful.

This meant that she had to assess God side by side with the magnitude of the promise.

- Does He have the ability?
- Does His have Integrity

  can He be TRUSTED?
- Does He have the resources
  [does He have what it takes]
- Is He Willing

- Was He faithful enough

- Can He be trusted

- Is He dependable

- Will He fail me

- Has He lied to me, will I be deceived

Sarah had to run a credibility check on God that is why it is said that "she judged Him faithful" the she concluded that God can be trusted.

It is only at this point that she believed and the Scripture says that she "received strength to conceive seed, and was delivered of a child when she was past age" Hebrews 11: 11

When she eventually believed, she was supernaturally enabled to take delivery of her promised seed.

Her faith activated the power within the promise to hand her the promise and she conceived and brought forth Isaac.

Where are you in your faith?

You must locate yourself in these two examples of great faith or no faith at all. We can tell if we have faith for something by our actions.

Sarah obviously could not believe what God had promised so she looked to her own solution, which was that her maid bare a child by her husband but when she truly turned and gave God a chance; her faith released the power, the ability of God inside the promise to deliver her child to her.

Now we sometimes think that we believe the Word of God or that we believe a promise of God, but we really do not because faith will make you do something that will activate the power within the promise.

You see the power of God is within the promise itself, the power is in the Word of God, and our ability to believe releases that power and puts it to work for us.

A while ago I had been asking God for a certain promise and after about five years, recently, in a time of prayer I brought the issue up and I heard in my spirit, the Lord said, "are you now ready" I was shocked because I thought I was ready all the while, and wondered why nothing seemed to be happening.

So, while I was asking, there was doubt in my heart because I was not yet ready for what I desired from God.

God knows us more than we do, we must be honest with God, let the Lord show us were we are at in our faith, and we can ask like the father whose son was torment by a demon of infirmity, we can cry out to Him and say, "Lord help my unbelief" help my inability to believe you at this stage.

God is faithful to help our faith when we are true to him and reach out for help. We will see how God helped Sarah

The prophecy

Is anything too hard for GOD? I'll be back about this time next year and Sarah will have a baby."

Genesis 18:14

The Angel made this affirmation of the ability of God to do absolutely anything for Sarah.

God knew that Sarah was overwhelmed with the staggering opposition in her body and she may not have had the confidence to put her faith on the line in case nothing happened we can all identify with this.

The Angel spoke the mind of God with an audacious authority with a finality that only God could exhibit and that sealed everything.

A timeline was eventually put in place [at the time of life – in nine month] for the fulfilment of this longstanding prophecy, and this helped Sarah to believe, it gave her something to hold unto, something to look to.

God can do the same for you too; "He is the same yesterday, today and forever" Hebrews 13: 8. He is a God that does not change. He says, "For I am the LORD, I change not" Malachi 3: 6

The Fulfilment of Prophecy

And the LORD visited Sarah as he had said, and the LORD did unto Sarah as he had spoken. 2 For Sarah conceived, and bare Abraham a son in his old age, at the set time of which God had spoken to him.

And Abraham was an hundred years old, when his son Isaac was born unto him. 6 And Sarah said, God hath made me to laugh, so that all that hear will laugh with me.

And she said, who would have said unto Abraham, that Sarah should have given children suck? For I have born him a son in his old age. 8 And the child grew, and was weaned: and Abraham made a great feast the same day that Isaac was weaned.

Gen 21: 1 - 8

God came down and helped Sarah's faith to receive her promise.

Now that is how faithful our God is. He will help you too if you will look to Him.

Since faith - which is our ability to believe God is required to see fulfilment of prophecy, our God who cannot lie will help our faith in His faithfulness, when we are struggling to believe, this is not the time to doubt and give up on God, but rather we can cry out to Him to help our faith.

He will help our faith so that we can believe Him and see His Word come to pass for us. If He did it before, then He will do it again, He is not a respecter of persons.

If we reach out to Him for help He will reach back and help us. He did it for Sarah; He will do it for you.

For the Scripture says:

I am crucified with Christ: nevertheless, I live; yet not I, but Christ lives in me: and the life which I now live in the flesh <u>I live by the faith of the Son of God, who loved me, and gave himself for me.</u>

Galatians 2:20

53

You do not have to wait any longer; the faith of Jesus is available to you, so reach out to God by the faith of our Lord Jesus Christ now.

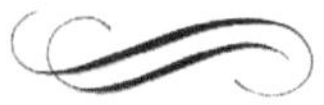

8

Jesus came to restore all things.

Jesus came to give us life

When **Adam fell**, sin came and with sin came death, but Jesus Christ the second Adam came and died to bring life to as many as will believe in Him and this life brings fruitfulness.

For if by one man's offence death reigned by one; much more they which receive abundance of grace and of the gift of righteousness shall reign in life by one, Jesus Christ.)

therefore, as by the offence of one judgment came upon all men to condemnation; even so by the righteousness of one the free gift came upon all men unto justification of life. 19 For as by one man's disobedience many were made sinners, so by the obedience of one shall many be made righteous. 20 Moreover the law entered, that the offence might abound. But where sin abounded, grace did much more abound:

21 That as sin hath reigned unto death, even so might grace reign through righteousness unto eternal life by Jesus Christ our Lord.

Romans 5: 17 - 21

We have already seen that our Lord Jesus came to die and pay a high price for the sin of mankind which is the birth place of all the affliction and oppression that we see around about us. He came to restore all things back to the way the Father wanted things to be. But this time in a more Glorious and intimate relationship with God because we have God Himself living inside us in the person of the Holy Spirit to perform His own counsel in our life.

For it is God which works in you both to will and to do of his good pleasure.

Philippians 2:13

Jesus came to give us life to overflow in every way if we can believe for it. Many are already living this abundant life today confirming that this life is available to us by faith.

God has revealed to us what His plan for us has always been and it says:

> For I know the thoughts and plans that I have for you, says the Lord, thoughts and plans for <u>welfare and peace and not for evil</u>, to give you hope in your final outcome.
>
> Jeremiah 29:11 – Amplified Translation

God's plan for you is welfare and peace and an expected end; these two words are very significant in their meaning and we will look briefly into them. Some translations say, "to do you good"

Therefore, we can say that; Peace, welfare with an expected end translates to "good" as God declared after He created everything in the Garden of Eden,

Welfare: noun [well and fare, a good faring]

1. Exemption from misfortune, sickness, calamity or evil; the enjoyment of health and the

common blessings of life; prosperity; happiness; applied to persons.

2. Exemption from any unusual evil or calamity; the enjoyment of peace and prosperity, or the ordinary blessings of society and civil government; applied to states.

Peace: Shawlowm – Original Hebrew text [Interlinear Bible]

> Completeness, soundness, welfare, peace
> Completeness (in number)
> safety, soundness (in body)
> welfare, health, prosperity
> peace, quiet, tranquility, contentment
> peace, friendship
> of human relationships
> with God especially in covenant relationship
> peace (from war)
> peace (as adjective)

Peace, well, peaceably, welfare, salute, prosperity, safe, health, peaceable,

Take the time to study what these words mean and it will give you a picture of what God's plan for you is.

Now it is not your responsibility to make this happen in your life, your part is to know and believe that this is what God wants for you.

Jesus said, "you will know the truth and the truth will make you free" Believe God and God will confirm His Word and bring His counsel to pass in your life as you walk with Him.

Many will argue that this life is not for us today but in the world to come, but the truth is that this is the life that Jesus came to give us now if we believe God for it. Faith comes by hearing and hearing by the Word of God.

What you know and believe is what you will be empowered to become John 1: 12.

Jesus always said, "be it unto you according to your faith" and He would say "according to your faith it will be done for you" so by your faith – that is your ability to believe the Word of God that comes to you like this one, you essentially determine the outcome of your life. It is always "according to your faith"

An expected end

The life of the believer is not uncertain, ours is not a game of chance or luck like the world system operates by, and God's plan for us is a secure and certain future.

We know what the future holds for us so we have hope and we can take our hope into the word of God and turn it to faith through the promises of God to us and we can receive what we desire now in this life

God sent His Son

How God anointed Jesus of Nazareth with the Holy Ghost and with power: who went about doing good, and healing all that were oppressed of the devil; for God was with him.

Acts 10:38

God anointed His Son Jesus with the Holy Ghost and with power and He went about doing "Good" Jesus went about doing the will of God which is called "good" that is what God sent Him to do.

He went about doing good and healing all that where oppressed of the devil for God was with Him.

God partnered with His Son Jesus to restore that Good that He wanted for man in the Garden of Eden.

Remember that at every stage of creation, "God said - and it was so – and God saw that it was good" God made everything "good" until sin came.

God sent His Son to come and restore all things back to Himself and as we believe, the Holy Spirit who is in us will do in us, for us and through us that which is pleasing unto the Lord. Philippians 2: 13

The Holy Spirit – One just Like Jesus

The Holy Spirit also came to carry on and continue the ministry of Jesus. The Lord said He is "another comforter" meaning one exactly like Himself, doing exactly like Jesus.

The Holy Spirit is the same Spirit that was working in Jesus and with Him to accomplish the plan of God and He is in us today to "will and to do" what pleases the Father.

Jesus said, "the Father in me, He doeth the works"

The Holy Spirit is that Spirit of the Father that worked in Jesus to fulfil the plan of God.

For God anointed Jesus Christ of Nazareth with the Holy Ghost and with Power who went about doing Good and healing all that were oppressed of the devil for God was with Him" Acts 10: 38

The Holy Spirit is that power of God that worked with and through Jesus during His earthly ministry to establish the plan of God, which is to do good and undo all the evil works of the enemy.

That Power of God is working in us today, just as if Jesus is with us because He is with us by His Spirit dwelling in us.

You may wish Jesus was here now and everything would be ok, but the truth as you know is that He is - the Holy Spirit is one exactly like Jesus doing the will of God inside the believer just as He did in Jesus

The Good news is that this time Jesus has died and God has raised Him from the dead and He is now sited at the right hand of the Father and guess with, you and I are sited with Him.

The Holy Spirit is working with us today exactly as He did with Jesus to establish the counsel of God for us and through us reaching out to all mankind.

As you receive your desires from God and have your needs met, you can reach out and become a partner with God by His Spirit to bring the same comfort to many.

In doing that Good and healing all that are oppressed of the devil as the Father partners with you through His Spirit. Glory to God!

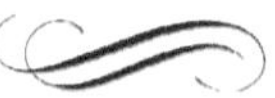

God partnered with His Son Jesus to restore that Good that He wanted for man in the Garden of Eden,

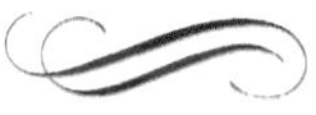

9

You must come into agreement

Agree with God

Just like the example of our father and mother Abraham and Sarah, we should do whatever it takes to come into total agreement with God, that is concerning what you desire from God and what He has provided in His Word that covers your desire.

Like Abraham, your faith can be in a place where you can instantly believe God and stand your ground irrespective of all the contrary and opposing circumstances that speak against the Word of God, and yet you believe anyway.

For Abraham "hoped against hope" and believed in hope. Like a servant of God said, Abraham "hope and then re – Hope" so after all hope was lost He still continued to hope any way. He believed anyway, so you must believe anyway irrespective of your situation or doctor's report.

Why did He have such a tenacious faith, was it because He just could believe God? No, we are told that He believed the God who had promised. That is the key to the kind of faith that brings results.

Abraham kept his eye on God and on what God had said, keeping your eye on God alone that is the key to faith that produces. *The faith that brings results does not believe today and doubt a little tomorrow, faith simply believes God and stays there.*

The difference with Sarah is that she considered the prevailing circumstance and so could not instantly come into agreement with God.

That is what prolonged things for years, she kept her eyes on the physical, she considered the impossible nature of her physical state and kept that in front of her and that hindered her faith until God returned and helped her faith.

The good thing is that when God helped her faith, she turned and came into agreement with

God and that removed the barrier of doubt and un-belief between her and her promised seed.

Agree with the Word

We must receive the Word of God and agree with the Word on Purpose. The Word of God is God. When God wants to do anything, He does it by His Word and by His Spirit.

Everything that we will ever need in this life is all deposited for us in His Word, if you want anything from God, don't look elsewhere just look to the Word. God will only confirm His Word and bring His own counsel to pass for us.

Go to the Word, run to the Word, receive the promise, believe it, make that promise your own because that is your title deed to that thing that you desire from God, the Word of God is your own portion in God so take it and make it your own and God is committed to fulfil it for you.

God requires your faith to do anything for you, the Word of God is the carrier and container of faith, the Word will produce for you the faith required to hand you that desired seed,

Position yourself to hear the word of faith eliminate every preaching that is contrary to what you believe God for, "because not all men have faith"

Reach out for messages of anointed servants of God that believe the Word of God and have testimonies in their life, then make sure you hear that preaching day and night.

It will eliminate doubt, and you will become fully persuaded and that is how you will come into agreement with the Word of faith to hand you your desired promise.

You must do all it takes to agree with the Word of God.

A servant of God making reference to the Word of God said recently, "the Kingdom of God suffers violence and the violent take it by force" and he then added "that is the force of faith" that is "violent faith" and I call this "Faith on purpose"

Come into agreement with your spouse

You must come into agreement with your spouse, be patient with one another. Sarah's faith was not in the same place with Abraham and it prolonged things.

The one with the stronger faith should gently with love strengthen the faith of the weaker spouse.

Pray together. Purposefully only talk to those around you who believe with you and others who do not, leave them out and walk in love in those relationships after all what you need is an agreement of two and the bond of Husband and wife is the strongest.

If a spouse finds themselves alone in their place of faith with the other partner not able to believe then the one with faith has the responsibility to find a covenant partner who will stand with them in faith until their desire comes to pass.

Remember that God helped Sarah's faith, He will help your too.

Prayer of Agreement

Again, I say unto you, that if two of you shall agree on earth as touching anything that they shall ask, it shall be done for them of my Father which is in heaven.

Matthew 18: 19

One of the most important and most powerful assets in the Kingdom of God is, praying in agreement or coming into agreement on any issue, Jesus said that the Father will do anything thing for us that we ask in a prayer of agreement.

This is an open check. He said, "as touching anything" this means that we are guaranteed 100% result and answer to prayer if we can simply find someone to genuinely stand with us in agreement on any issue of life that we are faced with.

Meaning that anything is possible and available to us on the platform of the prayer of agreement.

Prayerfully ask the Lord to lead you to the right person that can come into agreement with you.

Someone who believes in the fact that the promises of God are still for us today, someone who can commit to stand with you as an individual or with you as a family until your desire breakthrough is delivered to you.

God said that all it takes for us to have Him do anything whatsoever for us is to find someone, just one person to agree with us and we have our request granted.

This is an asset that we have not used very well in the body of Christ.

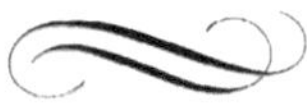

The faith that brings results does not believe today and doubt a little tomorrow, faith simply believes God and stays there.

"Having done all to stand"

Ephesians 10: 13 [Please read]

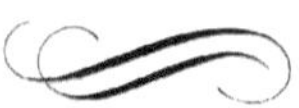

10

Final Word
How can this thing Be?

When the Angel came to Mary with the news that as a virgin she would conceive and give birth to a Son.

She asked him a vital question that answers for me and I believe for us all, how God will do.

"whatsoever we ask the Father in agreement" whatever our request maybe, the answers are the same today as it was the day that Mary asked the Angel this question:

Mary asked: How shall this be, seeing I know not a man?

The Angel answered giving us insight into how God works. He said:

This is the process: The Holy Ghost shall come upon you, and the power of the Highest shall overshadow you: therefore, also that holy thing which shall be born by you shall be called the Son of God. Luke 1: 35

This is the same order, this is how God does anything.

He sends the Word, and the Holy Spirit hovers over the surface and the power of God overshadows that situation and then the turnaround comes, that is, the breakthrough comes or in this case, conception takes place.

We find the promise, and we go to God in Prayer on the platform of His Word, then we believe we receive as we pray and the Holy Ghost hovers over the Word and brings it to pass for us in our area of need.

That is How God will do it: by His Word and by His Spirit and by your faith. Praise the Lord!

~~~
~~~

Have faith in God

Faith in God is the master key to a life of victory and triumph for us in the Kingdom of our God. Do whatever it takes to come to the place of absolute trust in God, persuade your heart to believe God, count on the integrity of God and in His Word.

Abraham was fully persuaded that God cannot fail Him, you can do the same.

The Scripture says that; even if we fail to believe, God abides faithful because He cannot deny Himself. God is faithful.

In Mark 11: 22, when the disciples witnessed that the fig tree that Jesus cursed had dried up the next day, they wondered and Jesus answered their amazement by giving us the key to doing mighty works and having breakthrough in life, He said "have faith in God"

If we believe not, yet he abides faithful: he cannot deny himself.

2 Timothy 2:13

You must come into complete agreement with God [that is with His Word] on any issue of life. God will partner with you by His Word and by His Spirit to hand you your desired breakthrough.

The Phrase "for God was with Him" has become for me a foundation for uncommon favour and mighty works.

Everyone that had this phrase mentioned with them had great victories in life, and we are in this category because God is with us.

~~~
~~~

The appointed time is now – not in the future

Faith is now, not in the future. We do not pray and hope that maybe God will answer or maybe someday God will come round and remember that someone was waiting somewhere for Him to move.

No, our faith moves God into action, we determine when God moves by our faith, our action and declaration of the promises of God in our area of need is what moves God into action in our behalf.

Some pray in hope and that is good because hope gives your faith something to work with.

But hope does not have the ability to hand you anything, rather hope enables you to hold unto the fact that your desire is possible, but hope cannot make it happen.

Because hope puts things in the future, but rather faith is now, faith is present.

It is your faith that will bring that desire into reality for you. You must take your desire into the Word of God find a promise for that desire and then receive it, believe it is for you.

Take it to God in Prayer, that is acting your faith and then the power will become available to give you your desired breakthrough.

By faith you determine what you want, when you want it, and how you want it, for "it is unto you according to your faith" and "it will be done for you as you have believed"

The Word of God is your guarantee and title deed to whatever you want from God. Find the promise, receive it, believe it, take it to God in prayer and it must come to pass for you, "it will be done for you as you have believed"

Faith is Now: NOW FAITH is the assurance (the confirmation, the title deed) of the things [we] hope for, being the proof of things [we] do not see and the conviction of their reality [faith perceiving as real fact what is not revealed to the senses]. Hebrews 11:1 – Amplified Translation

The time is Now: As God's co-workers we urge you not to receive God's grace in vain.

For he says;

- In the time of my favour I heard you,

- And in the day of salvation I helped you."
- **I tell you, <u>now</u> is the time of God's favour,**
- **Now is the day of salvation.**

  2 Corinthians 6:2 NIV

We pray to be answered now; our answer comes as we pray now, today not tomorrow.

Jesus said: Therefore, I say unto you, what things so ever ye desire, when ye pray, believe that ye receive them, and ye shall have them. Mark 11:24

It is when you pray that the answer comes on this side of Salvation.

It is not the same as the days of Daniel where the Prince of Persia withstood His prayer and it required Angelic reinforcement for his answer to come, no not today, because for us we have a seal, an authority, and a guarantee of our answer now that no demon in hell can withstand and that is the "wonderful – wonder working – miraculous - name of our Lord Jesus Christ.

The name of Jesus, the Authority of the believer

This is the authority of the believer. Jesus said before He ascended into Heaven;

And these signs shall follow them that believe; **In my name** shall they cast out devils; they shall speak with new tongues; 18 They shall take up serpents; and if they drink any deadly thing, it shall not hurt them; they shall lay hands on the sick, and they shall recover.

Mark 16: 17 – 20

That is the authority of the believer right there, so use it. A further guarantee that we have for answer to prayer and mighty works is the power behind that name and that is;

God also hath highly exalted him, and given him a name which is above every name: 10 That at the name of Jesus every knee should bow, of things in heaven, and things in earth, and things under the earth; 11 And that every tongue should confess that Jesus Christ is Lord, to the glory of God the Father.

Philippians 2: 9 -11

All the host of hell are now made completely subject to the name of Jesus Christ, so as we pray in faith by the authority of that name according to what God has said, then we have our desire granted us now.

Another major tool to answered prayer and having our needs met in prayer is praying according to the will of God which is praying according to the promises of God to us in His Word.

It is said that Abraham "believed according to that which was spoken, so shall your seed be"

He did not just believe that God can and will give him a child, but his faith was based on what God has said.

As we believe the promises of God and take it to Him in prayer, God is committed to confirm and establish it for us.

You hear a lot of believers say concerning a situation in their life "God will do it" Now that is verge, what is God going to do? What is the foundation of your faith?

Our faith must be based on what God has said in our area of need and nothing else.

The Scriptures say: God is not a man, that he should lie; neither the son of man, that he should repent: hath he said, and shall he not do it? or hath he spoken, and shall he not make it good? Numbers 23:19

What this implies is that. If He said it then He is committed to do what He has promised us in His Word.

Now Stop for a moment and settle in your heart that what you believe God for today is what He has said He will give you and then stand your ground.

If someone expects for me to buy them a car or pay their house rent and we have no relationship and I did not promise on any grounds to do those things for them, then I am not obligated to fulfil their desire.

They will be believing in vain because I did not promise it.

It is the same way with God, He is only committed and obligated to His Word and He watches over His Word to perform it for us.

He has raised His Word above His name; and His Word abides in Heaven for ever – so by all of this and so much more if you believe His Word, He can never fail you.

> And this is the confidence that we have in him that,
> if we ask any thing according to his will, he hears
> us:

> [15] And if we know that he hear us, whatsoever we ask, we know that we have the petitions that we desired of him.
>
> 1 John 5:14-15

What this scripture is saying is that if you pray based on assumption that "God will do it" as some are fond of saying, you will wait and wait.

Many experience delay in having their needs met because they are not diligent enough to settle down and ask the Holy Ghost to lead them to pray correctly for what they want.

You may think you are praying accurately but if your desire is not met, if your answer does not come - then seek the Holy Spirit to help you pray correctly.

Don't just assume that maybe God does not want to give me or maybe He wants me to wait, maybe it is not the right time.

We have added all of that to what God said. This is what He said, let us not add or remove from this:

> Again, I say unto you, that if two of you shall agree on earth as touching **anything** that they shall ask, it shall be done for them of my Father which is in heaven. Matthew 18:19

And in that day ye shall ask me nothing. Verily, verily, I say unto you, **whatsoever** <u>ye shall ask the Father</u> **in my name**, <u>he will give it you</u>. John 16:23

Therefore, I say unto you, **what things so ever ye desire,** <u>when ye pray,</u> <u>believe that ye receive them, and ye shall have them.</u>

Mark 11:24

Holy Spirit is our help in Prayer

But why pray based on assumption, why not go straight to the one who knows the mind of God concerning you in the first place.

He has access to the heart of God and can lead you to pray on target and your desire will come quickly as God desires for us.

In the same way, the Spirit helps us in our weakness. We do not know what we ought to pray for, but the Spirit himself intercedes for us through wordless groans. 27 And he who searches our hearts knows the mind of the Spirit, because the Spirit intercedes for God's people in accordance with the will of God.

Romans 8: 26 – 27 NIV

<div align="center">~~~</div>

The time of life:

The prophecy concerning the blessing of fruitfulness and conception always promised to deliver "according to the time of life."

So, if you have found the promise of God spend some time and build your faith. This is where the labour is, our labour is in the Word. And faith comes from the Word that we receive and believe and as faith comes it brings rest.

Faith comes with an assurance that produces peace and brings us into a place of rest, a quiet confidence in God and in His Word.

The Scripture says that Faith is our rest; we are to labour to enter that place of rest which is the place of faith that produces result.

As was suggested earlier, take messages that will help your faith, hear it again and again spend time in the Word of God until you are fully persuaded.

Then begin to say what you believe to yourself, say it to God in prayer, say it to the devil when doubt comes.

write it out and paste it all round your home and you will become fully persuaded beyond any kind of doubt.

As you do this, you have prepared the grounds for God to move on your behalf.

Remember this is a "day and night" affair and as we do this "we make our way prosperous and we will have good success" And again we are told:

> My son, attend to my words; incline thine ear unto my sayings. 21 Let them not depart from thine eyes; keep them in the midst of thine heart. 22 For they are life unto those that find them, and health to all their flesh.
>
> Proverbs 4: 20 - 22

■ Give attention to the Word of God in your area of need, put it in your eyes, in your ear and in your mouth, say it until you believe it, say it until it begins to talk back to you, say it until you become one with the Word, say it until you are fully persuaded and there are no more arguments in your heart with the Word, when the Word becomes flesh according to your faith, you will have it.

Keep it in front of you always and it will begin to form a mental picture for you so tangible that it will become physical in no time.

The Word is Spirit and everything was created by the Word of God, your baby and children will be conceived and born by the Word of God that says;

- "Be fruitful and multiply and replenish the earth" and as you believe this and do as we have said, this will become your reality now.
- To the shunamite woman, the Prophet said, "at the time of life"
- To Sarah the Angel of the Lord said, "at the time of life"

When your expectation has, a timeline attached to it, it will help your faith. It will help you to believe God more earnestly. So, do not be afraid to receive a timeline to what you desire after you have prayed.

I believe we ought to do this always.

Set a time line, Jesus said the timeline starts when you pray.

If you believe Jesus then you should expect the answer as you are praying, then thanks giving must precede answer to prayer.

All you must do after now is to spend time in quality thanks giving to God.

~~~
~~~

God will answer You speedily

Jesus said in Luke chapter 18 that even though the Father is more pleased with us when we use our faith, as a Father, He will also run to us as we cry out to Him ceaselessly.

God will respond to our unending cry of faith to Him.

> And shall not God avenge his own elect, which cry day and night unto him, though he bear long with them? 8 I tell you that he will avenge them speedily. Nevertheless when the Son of man cometh, shall he find faith on the earth?
>
> Luke 18: 7 - 8

Don't stop crying out to your Father, He will come to you and grant your desire.

Jesus also said that "If our earthly parents who are evil know how to give good gifts to us, how much more our Father who is in Heaven will not give "good things" to them that ask."

Before now He gives us a guarantee of answer to prayer, He said:

Ask, and it shall be given you; seek, and ye shall find; knock, and it shall be opened unto you: 8 for every one that asked receives; and he that seeks finds; and to him that knocked it shall be opened.

Matthew 7: 7 - 8

The psalmist also prayed to the Lord for urgent and speedy response to his prayer because of his desperate situation.

If you are in a desperate situation, you can also cry out to the Lord for a quick response to your prayer. After all the Lord has said that "he will do a quick work" so that His people do not become weary and fall away from the faith.

Hide not thy face from me in the day when I am in trouble; incline Your ear unto me: in the day when I call answer me speedily.

Psalm 102: 2

~~~
~~~

Do not forsake your Mercy

If you have any medical issues, take your healing and deliverance by faith according to the Word of God.

When you find the promise, and receive and believe it, as you keep declaring your faith, the creative healing power of God's Word will move to and fro in your system to heal and recreate anything that the enemy has stolen or brought into corruption.

I like the way the book of Jonah put it, He said: **There is mercy in God** so look to God and do not give up on God:

> They that observe lying vanities forsake their own mercy.
>
> Jonah 2:8

Here Jonah is calling any negative report "a lying vanity" he says that it is not real, if Jesus took it then you cannot have it, "for Himself took our infirmities and bore out sicknesses."

If the devil stole it then there is restoration, so either way, there is a solution in our God.

God will partner with you to bring that desired baby to you now. Acts 10: 38 [Read]

"How God anointed Jesus of Nazareth with the Holy Ghost and with power: who went about doing good, and healing all that were oppressed of the devil; for God was with him"

The Word of God is the truth that has prevailed over any fact.

Today during our family devotion, we spoke about this and my children gave their understanding about this and I promised to put it in the book.

- My son Joshua Jeremiah said: the truth changes the fact.

- My son Joel Alexander said: The truth will always prevail against the fact.

- Now Our Lord Jesus said: Sanctify them with the truth, Your Word is Truth. John 17: 17

- And Jesus said; You will know the truth and the truth will make you free. John 8: 32

The Word of God is that truth that prevails over every contrary situation in life. Acts 19: 20 Revelation 5: 5

Jesus is our mercy

I really want to point this out to you: If you say like those in the days that Jesus walked the earth, if you say, "Lord have mercy on me" I would like to let you know that – Jesus is our Mercy.

God has already had mercy on us by sending His Son to come and pay a high price for our Salvation which comes as a total package to restore to us those things that the enemy stole from us.

Blind Bathemaues said: Son of David have mercy on me

Jesus stopped and asked him: What mercy do you want? [paraphrase in mine]

Notice that he was prompt to answer "that I may receive my sight!

He knew exactly what he wanted without any iota of doubt.

- And Jesus straight away granted him that request because He Jesus is our mercy, He is the mercy of God sent to us, so do not forsake your mercy.

- Reach out and tell Him now what mercy you desire from Him and He is not a respecter of persons, He did it before, He will also respond to you now.

- This book is a gift of God to you to show you the mind of God for your fruitfulness so give God a chance, let Him partner with you now by His Spirit and by His Word to hand you your desire today.

~~~
~~~

You must forgive

Un-forgiveness is a major hindrance to faith and we know that faith is our purchasing power in this Kingdom. No matter what anyone has done to you, go ahead and forgive them

We are commanded to Love, and our faith will only work by Love.

If you harbour any kind of grudge, hate or resentment towards anyone even if they offended you greatly, to forgive that one is for your own benefit, so go ahead and forgive now.

If you find it hard, ask the Lord to help you and He will, remember He is in partnership with you to accomplish this assignment.

Un-forgiveness Jesus said is a snare of the devil, it is a pit he has dug for anyone to fall into, it is a trap so that he can steal, kill and destroy, so uncover this lie today and forgive.

Forgiveness is also an act of faith. You may not feel like it, faith is not a feeling anyway. Begin to declare to yourself that you forgive that person and are now walking in Love.

Soon enough it will become bearable enough for you to look them in the face and say it if necessary or at least you will no longer think about them and cringe inside you.

Use the tool of faith and declare that you forgive, that is faith by saying.

Remember the Master said, "if you will say to this mountain, be rooted up and be cast into the sea, it will be done as you have said" Mark 11: 23

Engage your power of faith by saying and come out of that hole, pit, snare, trap of the devil now

~~~
~~~

Receive the Spirit of Joy

In a devotional, recently a dear servant of God said that "one of the biblical words for joy is translated "to shine."

Another word means "to leap." Another means "to delight." But in every case, joy is more than an attitude, it is an action"

Joy is an outward expression of our confidence in our God.

Without Joy it is difficult to receive or take delivery of your inheritance in the kingdom of God. The Scripture says:

> Therefore, with joy shall ye draw water out of the wells of salvation.
>
> Isaiah 13:3

We need joy to draw from the Word of God which is the "well of Salvation" Joy is the tool that we use like a bucket that we can lower into the well of God's rich treasury of Salvation.

The Word of God contains all of our inheritance in Christ, and the Scripture is telling us that Joy is the way to draw from this rich treasury of God through Christ Jesus.

As a Source of power: Now Joy is one of the power sources of the Kingdom of God. For the kingdom of God is not meat and drink; but righteousness, and peace, and joy in the Holy Ghost. Romans 14:17

Without Joy: There is no fruitfulness, without Joy there is crop failure: Now read this and see the result of lack of Joy:

> The field is wasted, the land mourns; for the corn is wasted: the new wine is dried up, the oil languishes. 11 Be ye ashamed, O ye husbandmen; howl, O ye vinedressers, for the wheat and for the barley; because the harvest of the field is perished.
> The vine is dried up, and the fig tree languishes; the pomegranate tree, the palm tree also, and the apple tree, even all the trees of the field, are withered: **<u>because joy is withered away from the sons of men</u>**.

> **Joel 1: 10 – 12**

How will Joy come?

- By the Holy Ghost Romans 14: 17

- From the presence of God Psalm 16: 11
- As we praise and worship the Lord

Now as you praise and Worship your God, you are magnifying God above any contrary situation or report.

This also is an act of faith, you may not feel like it, but remember "faith has no feelings" faith is not about how you feel it is all about what God has said

When you worship your God, you are also provoking His manifested presence that brings about manifestation of our desire.

As you spend time to worship your God you take the focus off you and put is on your God. As you worship your God, you declare that, the situation is not your god.

You put God in His rightful place and He indeed will become God in that situation.

Everything will bow and give way to the plan of God to come to pass in your life, which is to "be fruitful and multiply and replenish the earth"

~~~
~~~

Take the Promise Now by the Spirit of Faith

Say what you want and it will be done for you as you have said – declare that you may be justified

The Woman with the issue of blood declared what she wanted from Jesus without involving Jesus in the process.

Jesus was only the point of contact for her faith to produce the result she wanted. For she said within her "if I may only touch the hem of His garment, I will be made whole"

She decided all by herself how her healing and deliverance would come and then she took it to the next level of faith which is action, she had a corresponding action to her faith.

She moved towards her solution. Mark 5: 23

The Centurion also called the shorts, after telling the Master the condition of his servant, he said to Jesus; you do not need to come into my house, I know how this thing works, "speak the Word only" and my servant will be made whole"

The Master was amazed at such great faith and gave him a blank cheque saying "it will be done for you as you have believed".

The Master called faith in the Word of God "great faith" Think about that, so we can put our trust completely in the Word of God and it will be done for us as we have believed Matthew 8: 5 - 13

Now how have you believed so that "it will be done for you as you have believed" the Master gave us this guarantee.

So now the ball is in your court, the Father has come to help your faith.

Do you believe that in nine to ten months from reading this book and believing?

That is being fully persuaded that it is the will and plan of God for you to be fruitful and multiply and replenish this earth irrespective of what has happened in your life or your body, irrespective of the time that we now live in.

If you believe this without an ounce of doubt, then you must put your faith out there and declare yourself pregnant. Or declare your wife pregnant to bring to birth in the next nine to ten months from when you have read this book over and over again until you are fully persuaded. And "judge God faithful who has promised." And then you will certainly take your own promised seed.

Jesus asked the two blind men that came to desiring mercies of Him a fundamental question.

I want you to take your time to answer this question as though Jesus was asking you.

Answer for yourself and you will get the same response from Jesus right now, because, "He is the same yesterday, today and forever"

He said, "I am the Lord and I change not" Now answer this:

Two blind men crying said to Jesus: Thou Son of David, have mercy on us.

Jesus to the blind men: Do you believe that I am able to do this?

The two blind men respond: Yes, Lord.

Then touched he their eyes, saying; According to your faith be it unto you. Matthew 9: 27 - 31

The spirit of faith speaks

The Psalmist said: I believed, therefore have I spoken Psalm 116: 10a

And on this side of Salvation: We having the same spirit of faith, according as it is written, I believed, and therefore have I spoken; we also believe, and therefore speak; 2 Corinthians 4: 13

What do you say now?

You must say what you want to see and not what you see.

The Woman with the issue of blood said what she wanted "if I may but touch --- I will see" she kept saying to herself "if I touch --- I will see"

What do you say and keep saying to yourself?

Declare your faith by saying:

- The Blessing is upon me through Christ Jesus
- For I belong to Christ; therefore, I am the seed of Abraham and an heir according to the promise,
- I have inherited the blessing of my father Abraham – therefore I am fruitful and I multiply and replenish the earth as the Holy Spirit hovers over me and the power of the Highest over shadow me.
- I now conceive seed to bring forth my son or daughter.

In the Wonderful miracle name of our Lord Jesus Christ,

Galatians 3: 13 – 14. Galatians 3: 29.

Now declare to your body: "I command my body to get in line with God's Word and function perfectly, and I demand that my body receive and produce seed as a baby now in Jesus' Name".

~~~
~~~

Now I pray for You

Prayer of agreement:

Our Point of contact: Again, I say unto you, that **if two of you** shall agree on earth as touching anything that they shall ask, it shall be done for them of my Father which is in heaven. KJV

When two of you get together on anything at all on earth and make a prayer of it, my Father in heaven goes into action. Matthew 18:19 –MSG

I Pray for you and come into agreement with you: Father Lord based on your Word, I set myself in agreement with this your precious child that as you asked in Genesis 18: 14

"Is there anything too hard for the Lord" and again Lord You said in Jeremiah 32: 27

"I am the God of all flesh, and there is nothing too hard for me"

Now Lord You also said that we should ask anything in the name of our Lord Jesus and we shall receive, that our Joy maybe full"

It is your desire that the Joy of your children be full therefore, we now ask that you grant that this your child who is a seed of Abraham find joy and fulfilment as they receive their desired seed.

Let the wife become pregnant at the instance of this prayer and bring forth their desired seed at the time of life as You have said in Genesis 18: 14.

Father return at the time of life and visit this family and confirm your Word, Lord let their Word come now to the praise of our Holy name.

By stretching forth Your hand to heal; [to bless, deliver, restore, create] Lord let creative miracles take place now where necessary and that signs and wonders may be done by the name of Your Holy Child Jesus. Acts 4:30

Mighty Holy Spirit, Lord hover over this your child, restore order to the entire system, cause every hormone and chemicals in the body to line up with your command that we be fruitful and multiply and replenish the earth right now.

Mighty God, cultivate the womb and prepare it for conception now, in the miracle working name of our Lord Jesus Christ.

Let the power of the Highest come upon and overshadow to cause conception to take place right now.

Mighty God supply the strength as you supply the faith and let your word come at the time of life to bring forth the fruit of a child to this family, to the Glory of Your Holy name.

Thank you, Blessed Lord, and we return all the Glory to you. In the name of your Son our Lord Jesus Christ

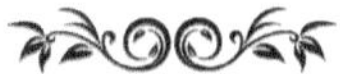

If this book has been given to you as a gift and you do not already know Jesus as your Lord and saviour, now is the perfect opportunity to do so.

You see, only as a child of God through salvation in Jesus Christ will you benefit from the terms of this covenant – that is everything that is written in this book which is all based on the Word of God. The scriptures say that;

> Neither is there salvation in any other: for there is none other name under heaven given among men, whereby we must be saved. And Romans 10:13 says; "For whosoever shall call upon the name of the Lord shall be saved."
>
> Acts 4:12

This is how we all get saved by faith

That if thou shalt confess with thy mouth the Lord Jesus, and shalt believe in thine heart that God hath raised him from the dead, thou shalt be saved.

10 For with the heart man believeth unto righteousness; and with the mouth confession is made unto salvation. Romans 10:9.

Pray this prayer and believe.

Father I confess with my mouth That Jesus Christ is Lord and I believe in my heart that you raised Him from the dead. Lord Jesus I open my heart to you, come into my heart and become my Lord and saviour, forgive all my sin and accept me now into your kingdom, Lord fill me with your Holy Spirit.

I receive salvation now and I receive your wonderful gift of the Holy Spirit in Jesus name, Amen.

Please note: It does not stop there, after we receive Jesus as our Lord and saviour, we must get into fellowship with the brethren, so ask the Lord to lead you to the right place of fellowship and especially get a good Bible and Christian books and messages to build your faith as we have heard in this material to enable your growth and spiritual understanding. Finally, I commit you to God and to the Holy Spirit, as it is written: "And now, brethren, I commend you to God, and to the word of his grace, which is able to build you up, and to give you an inheritance among all them which are sanctified." Acts20: 32. Be Blessed!

~~~~
~~~~

About Heavenly Life Worldwide Missions

We are a ministry in response to the instruction of our Lord Jesus Christ in;

Mat 28: "All power is given unto me in heaven and in earth. 19 Go ye therefore, and teach all nations, baptizing them in the name of the Father, and of the Son, and of the Holy Ghost: 20 teaching them to observe all things whatsoever I have commanded you: and, lo, I am with you always, even unto the end of the world. Amen."

Also in Mark 16: Go ye into all the world, and preach the gospel to every creature. 16 He that believeth and is baptized shall be saved; but he that believeth not shall be damned. 17 And these signs shall follow them that believe; in my name shall they cast out devils; they shall speak with new tongues; 18 they shall take up serpents; and if they drink any deadly thing, it shall not hurt them; they shall lay hands on the sick, and they shall recover.

We do this through the following platform:
- The Working Document – Book Publishing
- Media – Network Broadcast
- The feed my Lamb Project/Foundation

Small Business Finance and Education Scholarships.
- Weekly and monthly Community-wide distribution of Gospel Tracts and Bibles

Our true Heritage in Christ Jesus can only be found in the Word of God, as it is written: "And now, brethren, I commend you to God, and to the word of his grace, which is able to build you up, and to give you an inheritance among all of them which are sanctified. Acts 20:32
Jesus Christ is Lord Forever!

~~~~
~~~~

ABOUT THE AUTHOR

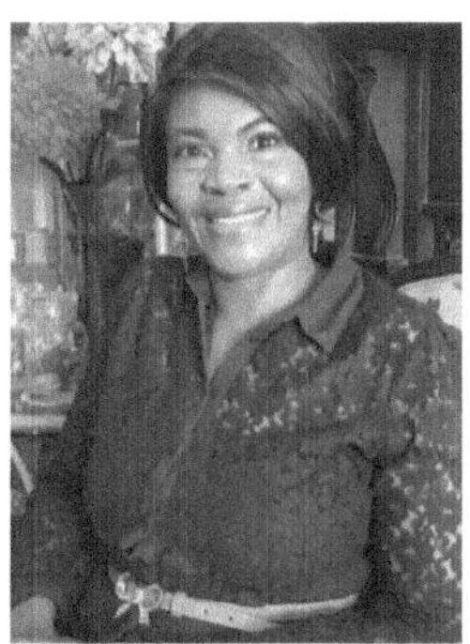

Margaret Ema

Margaret Ema is serving the Lord Jesus in ministry in a World missions outreach and in the marketplace according to Matthew 21: 6 - 7 She is Host of Heavenly life missions Worldwide. Margaret serves the Lord in Media and Publications, as a Business Consultant, Entrepreneur, Conference speaker. She holds a BSc Hons in Digital Technology, Innovation and Creativity. Dublin Institute of Technology. A Post Graduate Cert in International Management, Liverpool University. UK.

Main Focus: Mentorship

She is a mother of four lovely boys.

Other titles from Margaret Ema:

- **Books in Collections.**

  Books in All Formats - Print. EBook and Audio.

1. Faith – Breakthrough Collection.
    - Let Jesus Show you how to Use your Faith on Purpose.
    - Use Your Faith on Purpose.
    - Faith in God.
    - You must Fear no Evil

2. Healing and Health Collection.
    - Holy Spirit, the Healer Within You.
    - Healing and Health – Your Health Care Package.
    - Health and Cure quick Read.
    - Healed by the Miracle Hand of God.

3. Business and Money.
    - Release of Wealth – Wealth in Troubled times. COMING SOON!
    - The Power of the Blessing. COMING SOON!
    - The Access Code. COMING SOON!

4. Success Collection
    - Dare to Ask. COMING SOON!
    - Just Dot It. COMING SOON!
    - 7 Pillars of Success. COMING SOON!

5. Living in the Supernatural Collection.
    - God inside You – Unlimited Capacity.
    - Living now in the Realm of God.
    - We dwell in Light. – Understanding your Advantage in Life.

6. Family Success.
    - Marriage – Enjoyment not Endurance – A practical Handbook.
    - Marriage – Build according to pattern – Live by Design.
    - Naked and Not Ashamed.
    - Miracle Baby.

7. Creating your World.
    - **Let there be light - Create your World**
    - **Morning Glory**

Email ME at: connect@heavenlylife.org

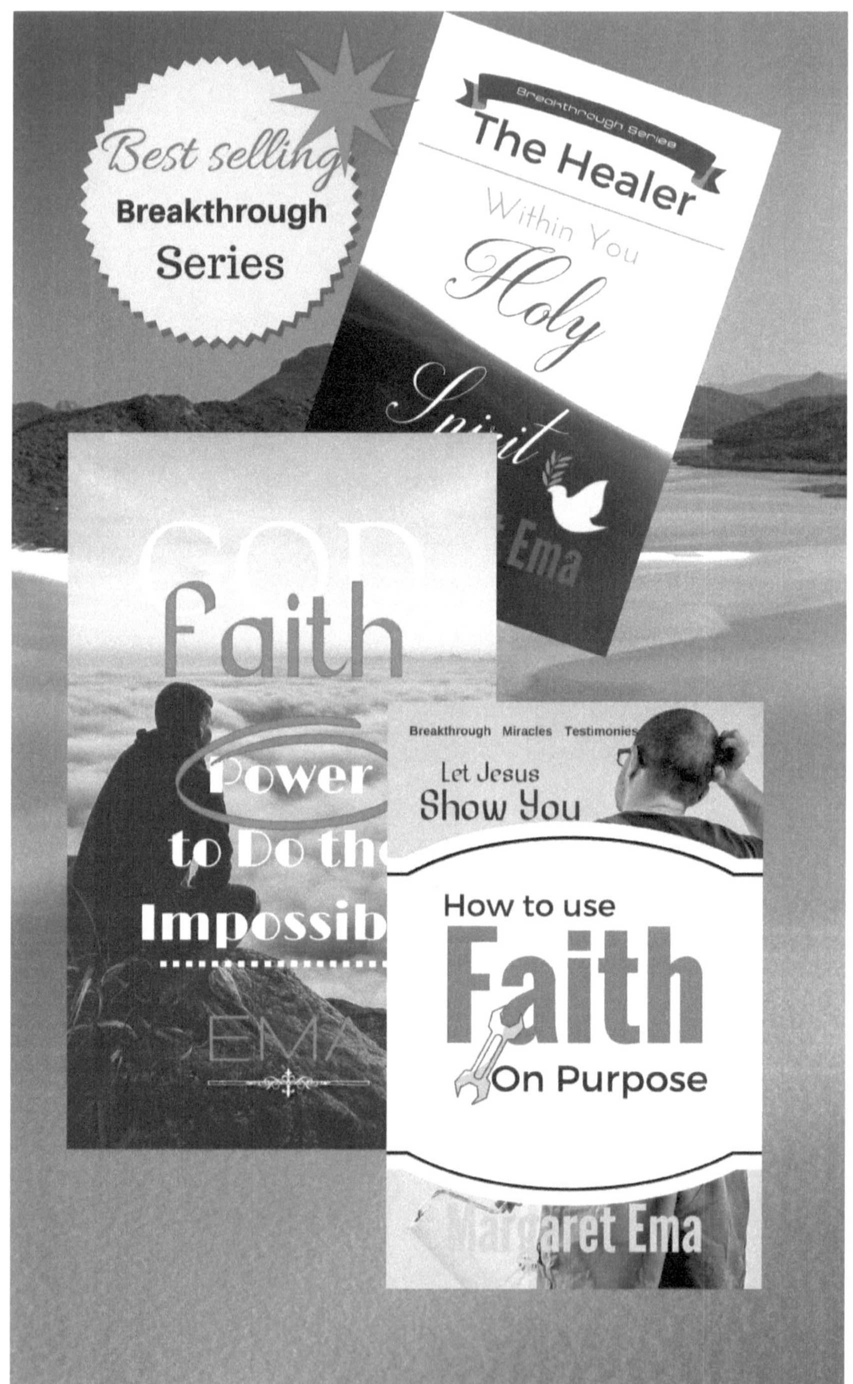
Best selling
Breakthrough
Series
Breakthrough Series
The Healer
Within You
Holy
Spirit
Ema
GOD
Faith
Power
to Do the
Impossib
EMA
Breakthrough Miracles Testimonies
Let Jesus
Show You
How to use
Faith
On Purpose
Margaret Ema

Work Book

Notes

Notes

Notes

Notes

Notes

Notes

123

Notes

Notes

125

Notes

Notes

Notes

Notes